TESSIE AND NESSIE
GO TO THE
SPA

Shekhar and Company
An illustration company focused on the children's industry.
shri8384@gmail.com

For Nessie, a girl
who lost weight by exercising
and eating right
and
Tessie, a horse
who loved her.

Tessie was a horse. Sometimes she didn't think she was a horse, but she lived on a farm and loved to run in the fields. She said, "neigh" and "phwwwwww" and occasionally "nicker" and "whinny". She had a long nose with a white stripe and four legs, three with white socks, and hooves.

All the other horses liked playing with her. She liked galloping around the field, tossing her head and neighing to the other horses. She liked to eat oats and hay and snacks of apples and carrots, but her favorite food was grass. She liked kicking up her heels in Spring. She liked dew drops on flowers and whiskers on other horses' noses, and running very fast.

She was probably a very nice horse, don't you agree? (You can answer questions in this book by saying "yey" meaning "yes" or "neigh" meaning no in horse talk or any way you want to.) This book is about losing weight but "wait", don't worry, if a horse can do it so can you.

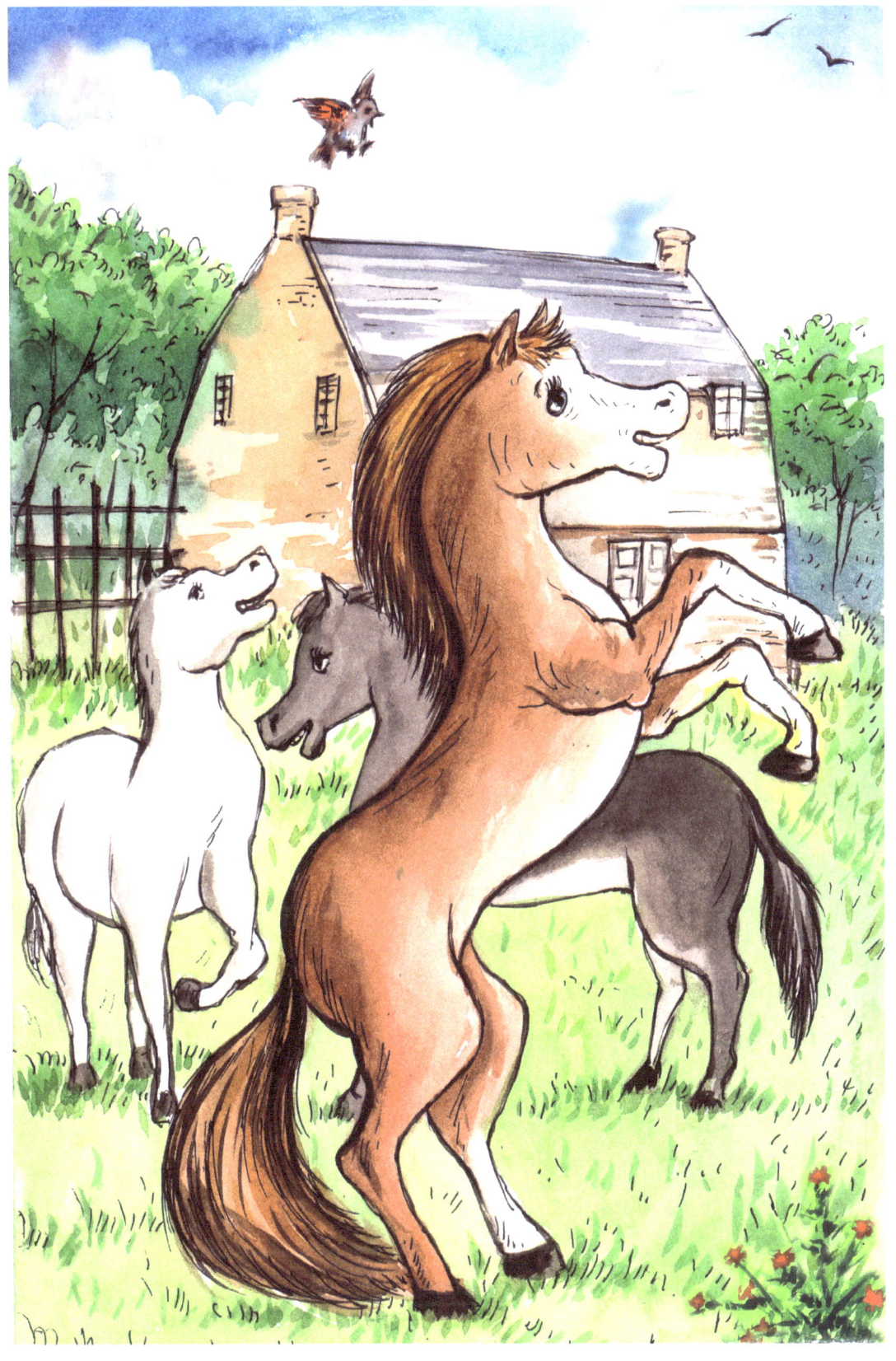

Vanessa was an nine-year old girl with long chestnut-colored hair like Tessie. She lived on the same street as Tessie but in a house with her parents and her brother. She couldn't really neigh, although she liked to try because she loved horses, especially Tessie. Sometimes she even thought she was a horse. Vanessa often walked down the street to the farm where Tessie lived and fed her apples or carrots. The stable manager told her not to give Tessie sugar or candy because it was not good for horses.

Her best friend, Amy, lived across the street, and they studied together, went to movies together and played soccer together. Vanessa loved playing with Amy. Sometimes they pretended to be horses and neighed and ran around the yard. They also liked eating snacks while they were doing their homework.

Do you ever pretend to be a horse or another animal that you like?

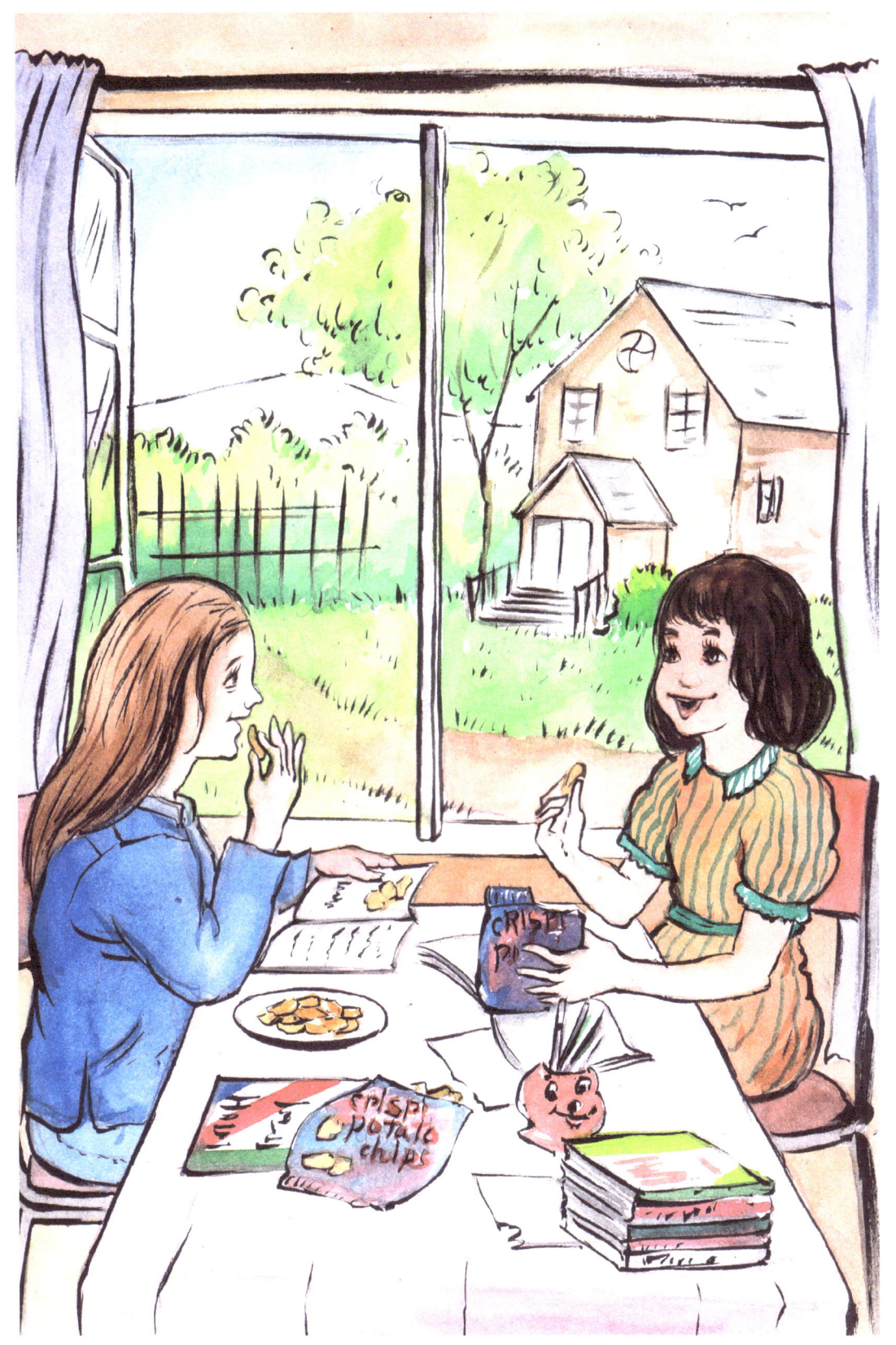

In the spring it rained and rained. The girls couldn't go outside and play because of the rain and mud. They had to sit around the house after school, and they couldn't think of anything to do when their homework was finished except eat and watch television.

Tessie could go outside, but the grass in the field had grown very long because of the rain. Tessie ate way too much of the tasty green grass. She gained so much weight that her ankles began to hurt, and she couldn't run in the arena or even walk around the barn. The veterinarian said she had a hoof problem, and it was serious! She had to stay in her stall with her hooves in a bucket of ice and take medicine. The other horses stared at her and snorted. It sounded like they were laughing at her. Then even her friends stopped visiting her at the barn door.

Poor lonesome Tessie! Did you know horses could eat too much just like people?

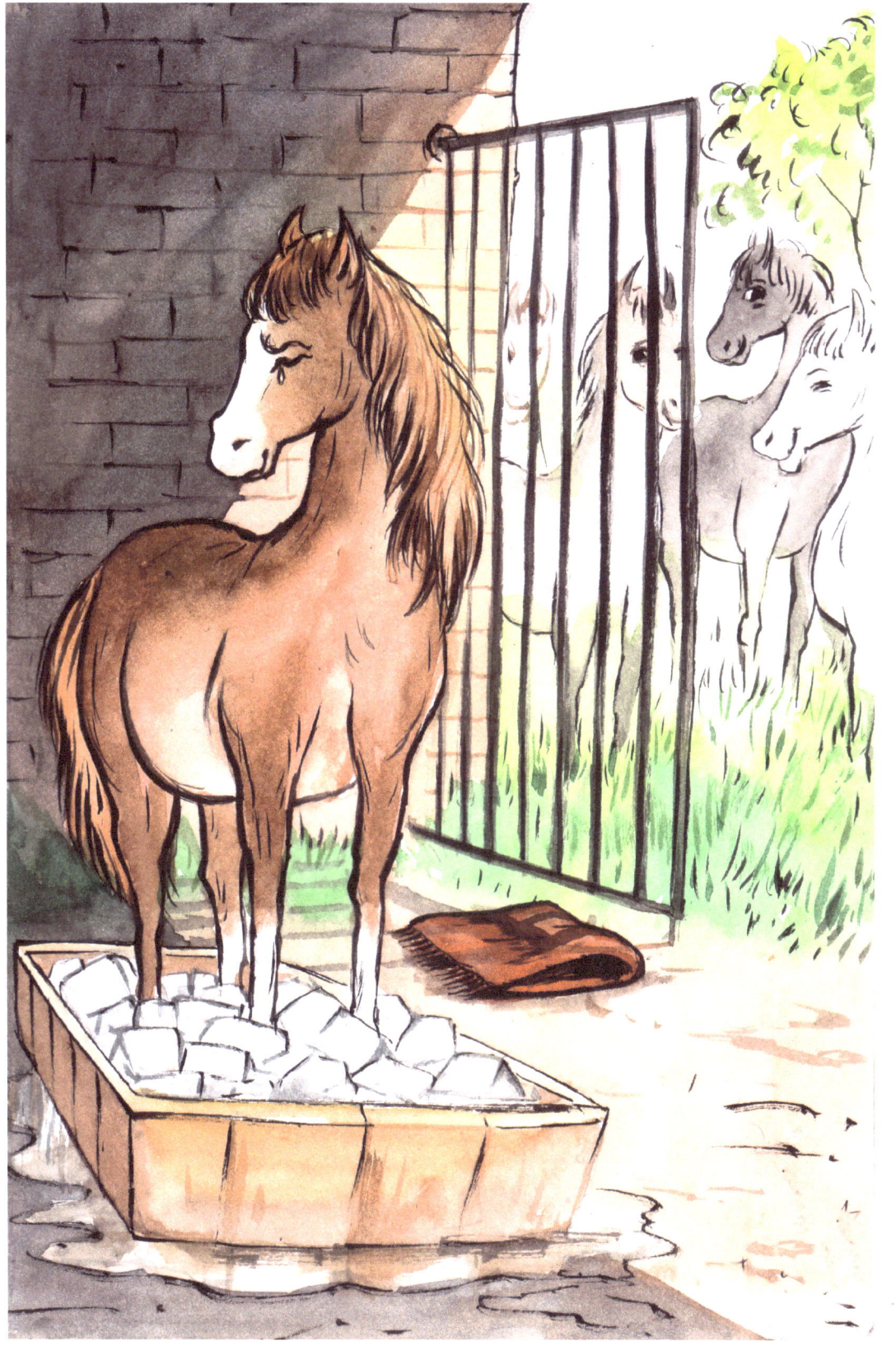

Vanessa was already very unhappy because of the rain, and then one day Amy came over to say that she was moving away. Vanessa felt very sad and lonely and started hanging out with banana splits, popcorn, candy, and cookies. She began to gain weight and couldn't play soccer very well because she couldn't run fast. Her clothes didn't fit, and her brother started calling her Nessie because she looked kind of large around the middle like the Loch Ness monster.

The Loch Ness monster is a legendary dinosaur-type creature that may live in a lake in Scotland. It is seldom seen because it dives under water when people are around. Vanessa dove for her bedroom whenever her brother's friends came in the house, just like the Loch Ness monster. She might have been eating too many snacks because she was bored and lonesome and didn't want to be seen because she was gaining some weight.

What do you think caused her to eat too much, and what kind of snacks do you eat?

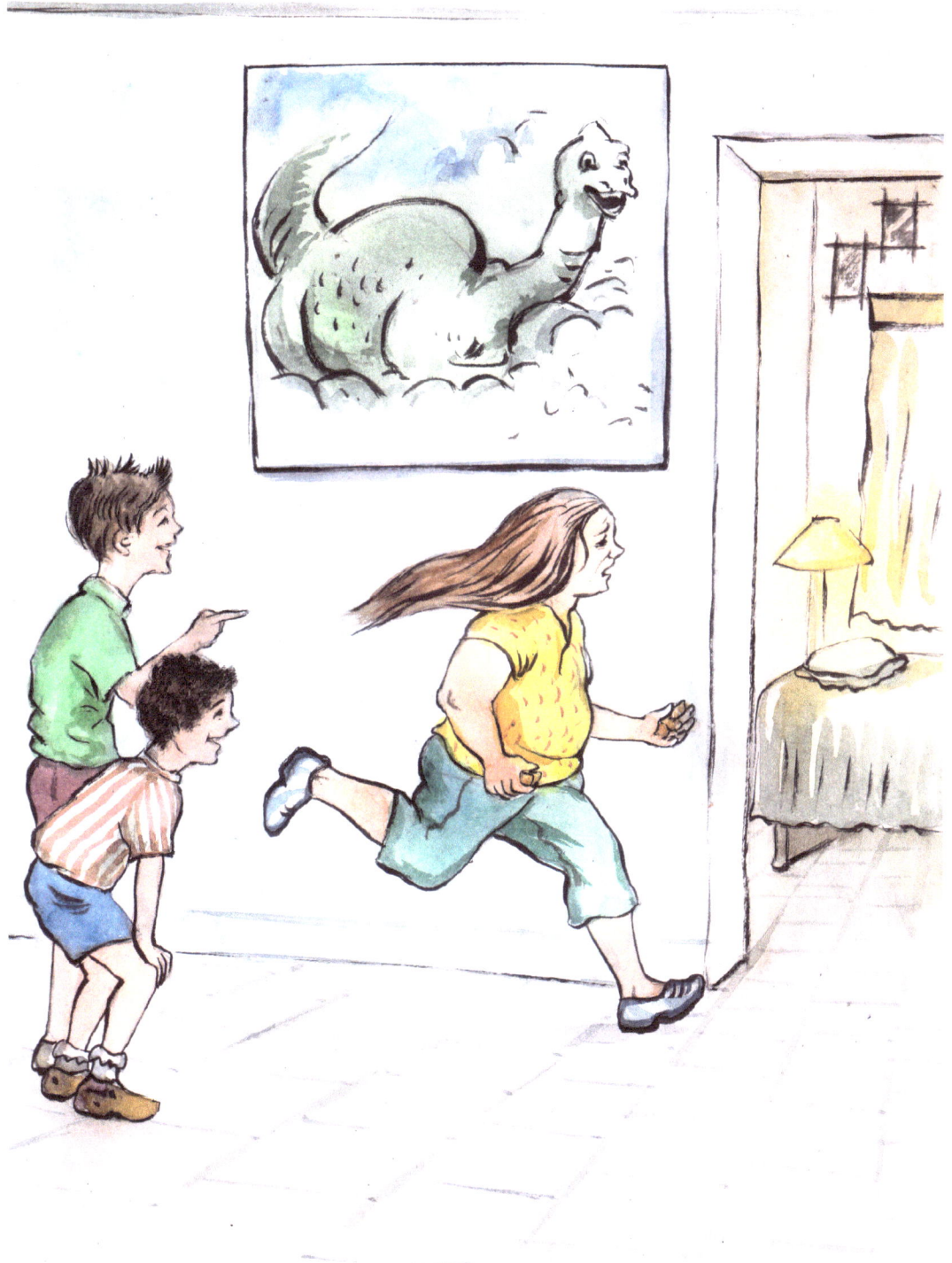

Finally it stopped raining, the sun came out, and Nessie hurried down to the farm where Tessie lived. She didn't see Tessie outside so she asked the stable manager where Tessie might be. He said, "Tessie has eaten too much grass and has to stay in her stall until she loses weight so she won't hurt her feet." She is grounded. Nessie had been grounded before too and didn't like it. She tried to think about how she could help Tessie.

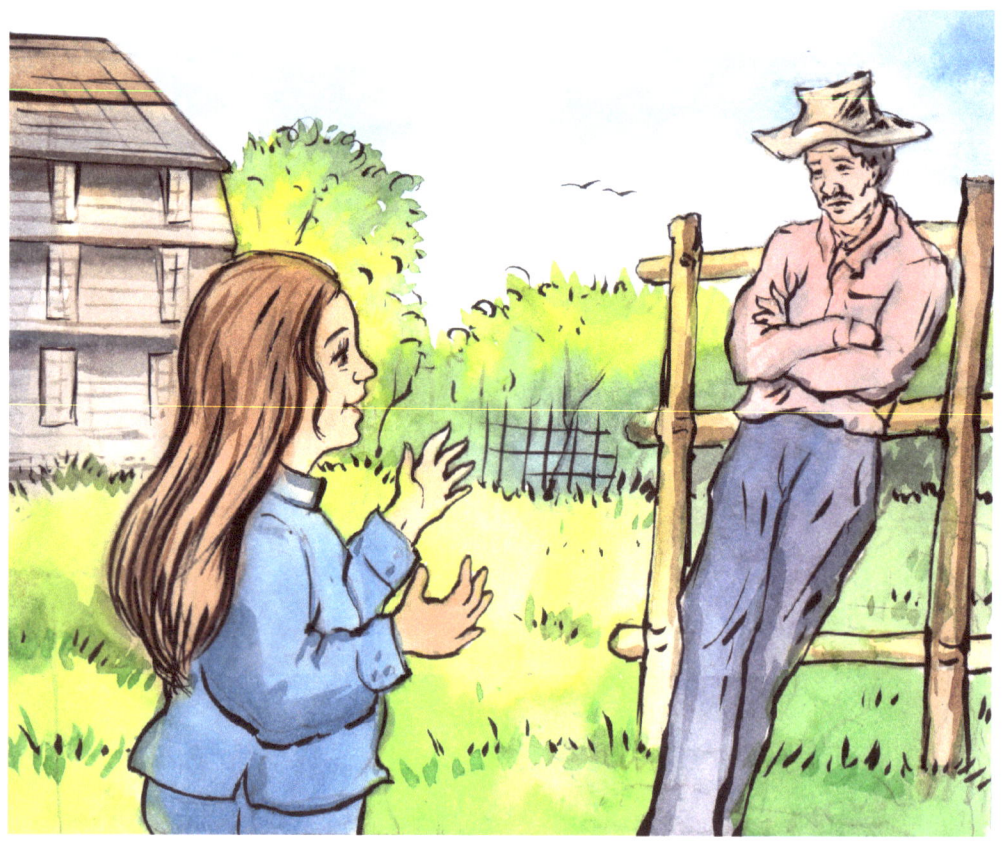

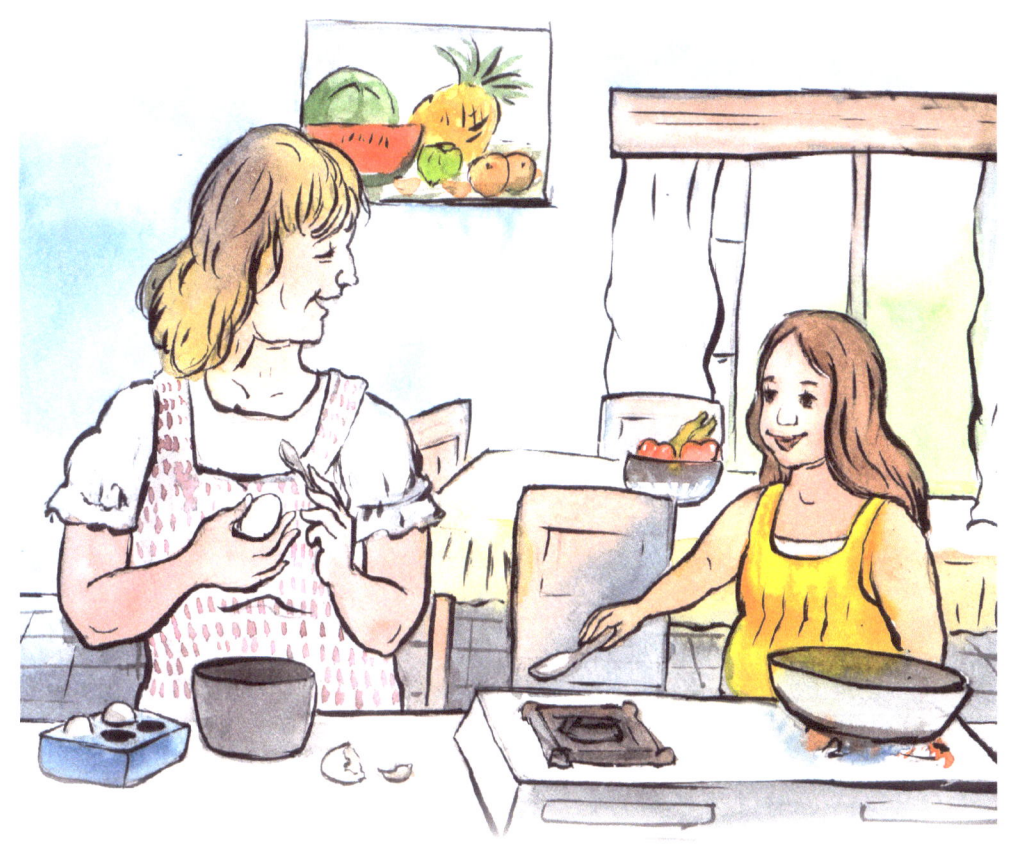

When she got home she asked her mother if she could take horseback riding lessons. Her mother said, "I thought maybe you would like to go to the gym with me, but I know how much you love horses. If you help with the dishes and some chores around the house you can take lessons." Nessie had a nice mother, don't you think?

Does your mother help you think of ways to get some exercise?

That night Nessie's mother ordered pizza for dinner because it was her brother's birthday. Nessie ate only two pieces at the table with her family since her brother was watching. But she tiptoed back into the kitchen after everyone had gone to bed and quietly opened the refrigerator door. There was a whole pizza left, and she took it back to her bedroom. She got under the covers with her flashlight and ate pizza and read her favorite book about horses.

She learned that horses sometimes eat too much grain or rich grass and gain weight, which causes their ankles to swell. This is often very painful for horses, and they aren't able to walk or even stand in their stall. She also read that lack of exercise might make the condition called "laminitis" even worse. Nessie was so busy reading that before she knew it, she had eaten the whole pizza.

She was probably worried about Tessie, but do you think it was a good idea to eat so much pizza right before going to bed?

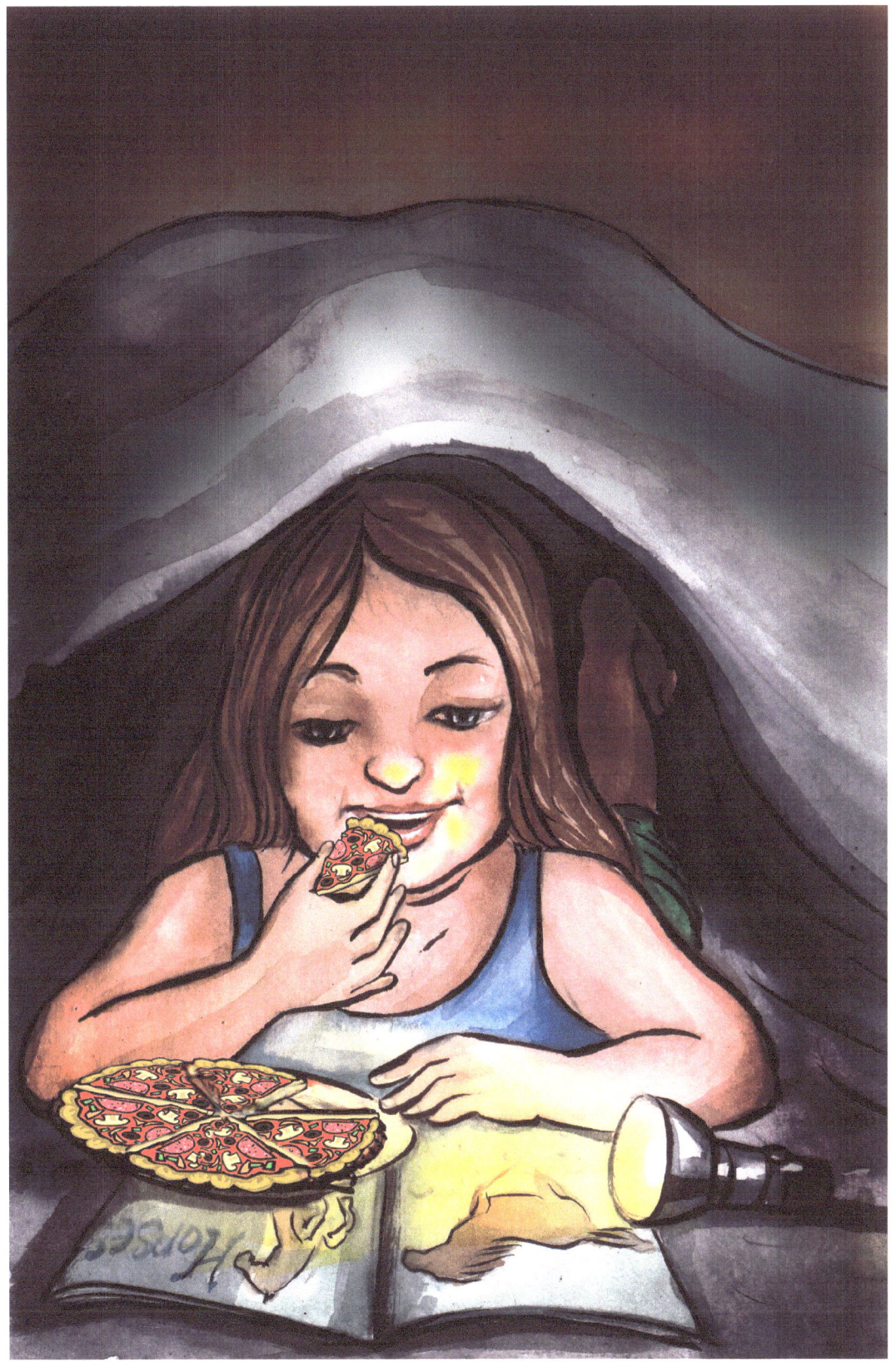

Nessie was surprised at how quickly the next morning arrived, and she was at the horse farm. Tessie was neighing to her loudly from the barn and Nessie could understand every word she said. She said, "Heeehehehehehehehehehehelp, Heeehehehehehehelp, Heehehehehehehehelp!" Nessie said, "Don't worry Tessie. I will help you. Maybe you can come with me to my mother's health spa and gym to get back into shape." Tessie said "yey," and away they went to buy a jogging suit.

Nessie tied Tessie to a lamppost by the mall and said, "Wait here while I get you some workout clothes." She came back with an extra extra extra extra large jogging suit in green and red to go with Tessie's chestnut-colored hair. Tessie reared up and neighed loudly while Nessie pulled and pushed and twisted and yanked until she got the suit on Tessie. They were both sweating and felt like they already had quite a workout.

Do you think it is easy to put a jogging suit on a horse?

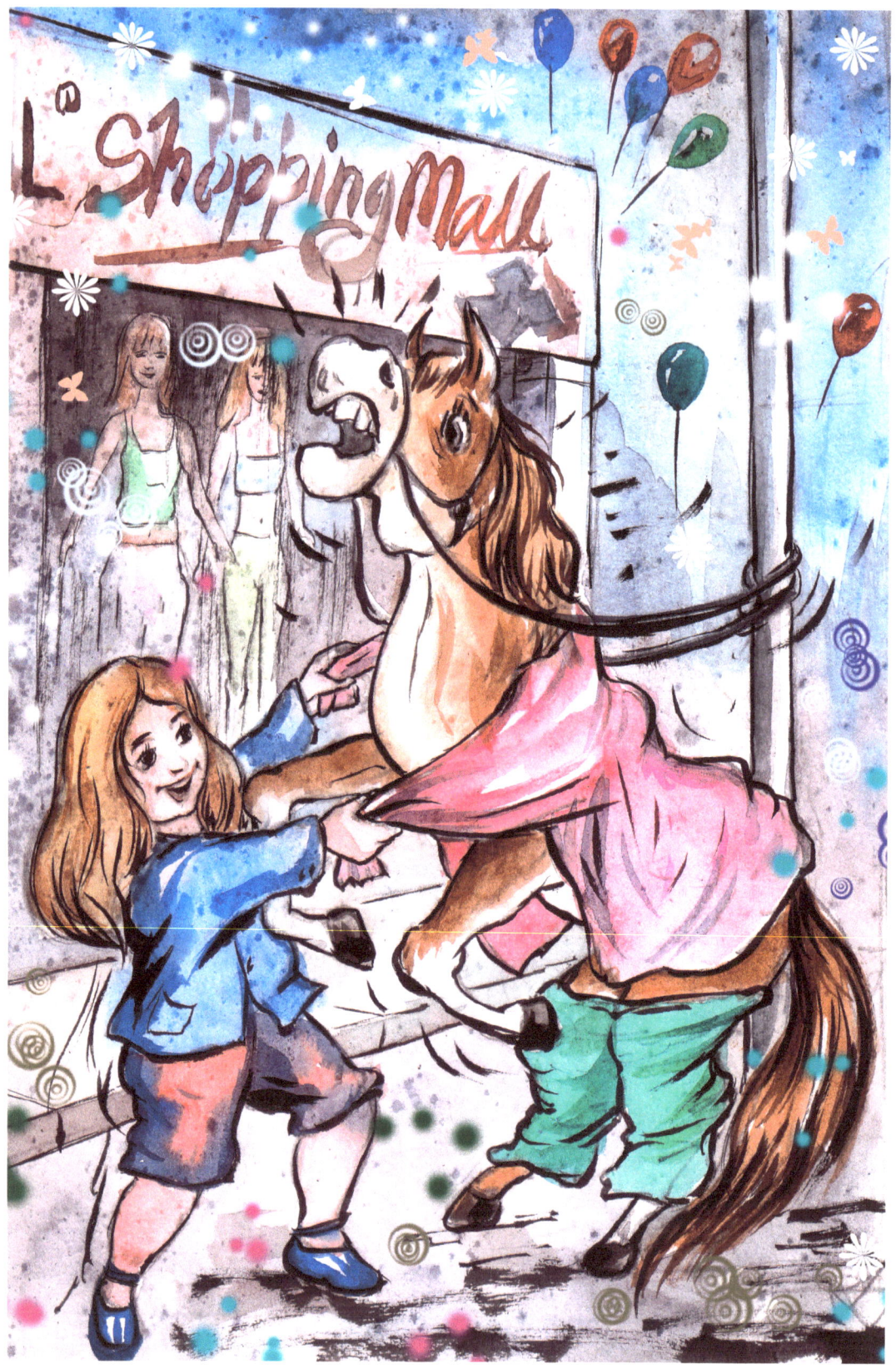

When they entered the spa, they met Bessie Biceps. She said she was their teacher and was glad to have two new students. She started the treadmill machine for Tessie. Tessie liked it at first, but Bessie kept turning it up faster and faster.

Soon Tessie was

trotting,

then cantering,

then galloping!

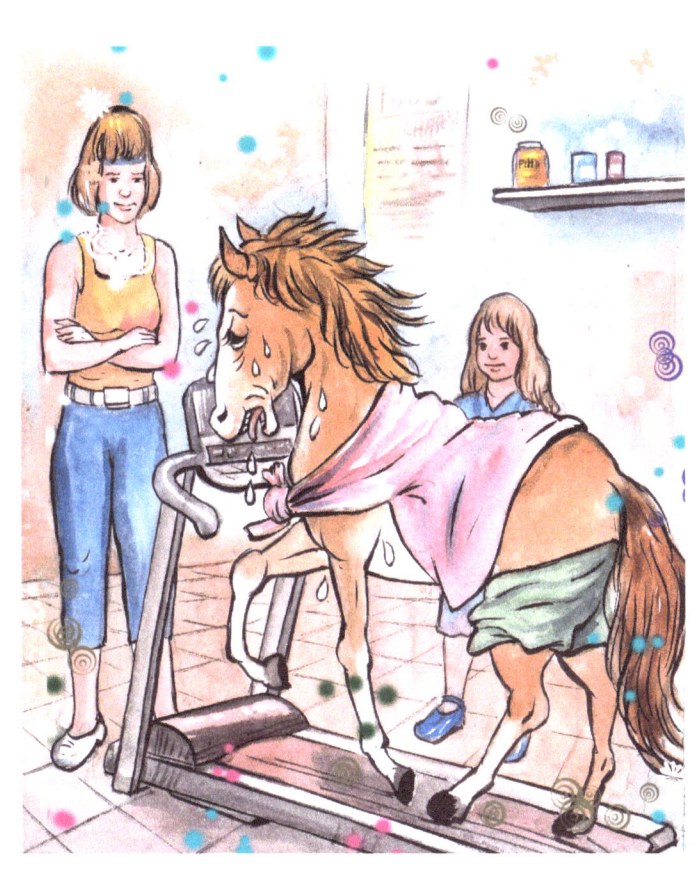

As soon as she began to gallop, she crashed right through the wall above the fine restaurant by the pool. Tessie looked like a moose mounted on the wall to the well-dressed diners below. The handlebars from the machine were her antlers.

Sounds pretty silly, don't you agree?

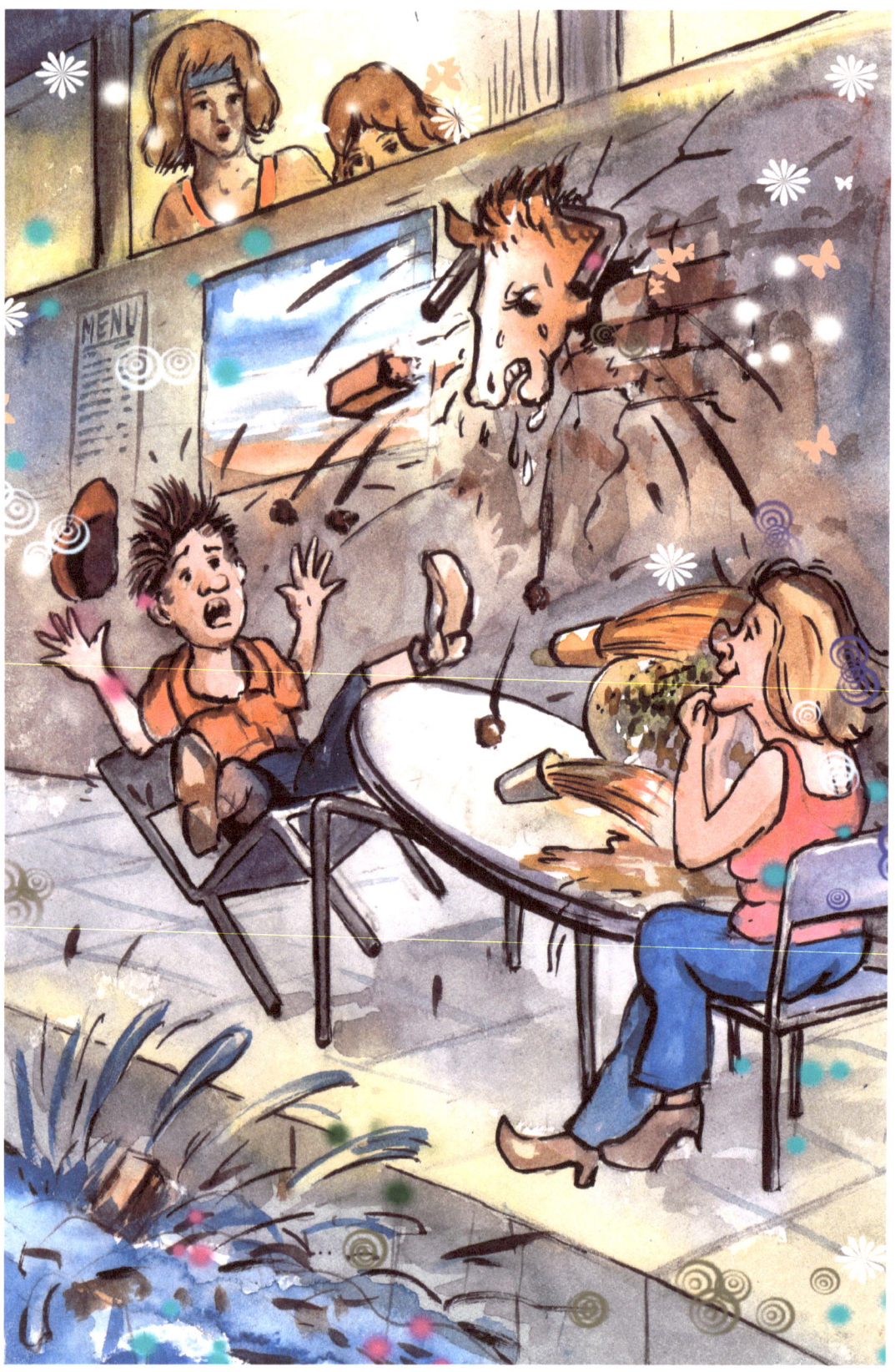

Bessie was a little surprised but impressed none-the-less. She pulled Tessie back by the tail and took her to the weight lifting machine. Tessie sat down on the seat, but she was so heavy that the machine crunched to the floor, and the weights went flying everywhere.

Bessie sighed, "I have never had a customer like this. She weighs as much as a horse." Nessie tried to tell Bessie that Tessie *was* a horse, but Bessie wasn't necessarily listening. She didn't seem to notice that Tessie had four feet and neighed. She was more interested in how much she weighed.

She led Tessie and Nessie to the sauna. "Maybe they need to sweat off a few more pounds before they try the equipment," announced Bessie to the towel lady. Bessie gave them towels and let them sit on the wooden seats next to the hot rocks and shut the door. The sauna is very hot and makes people sweat. It felt good for a while, but soon it got too hot.

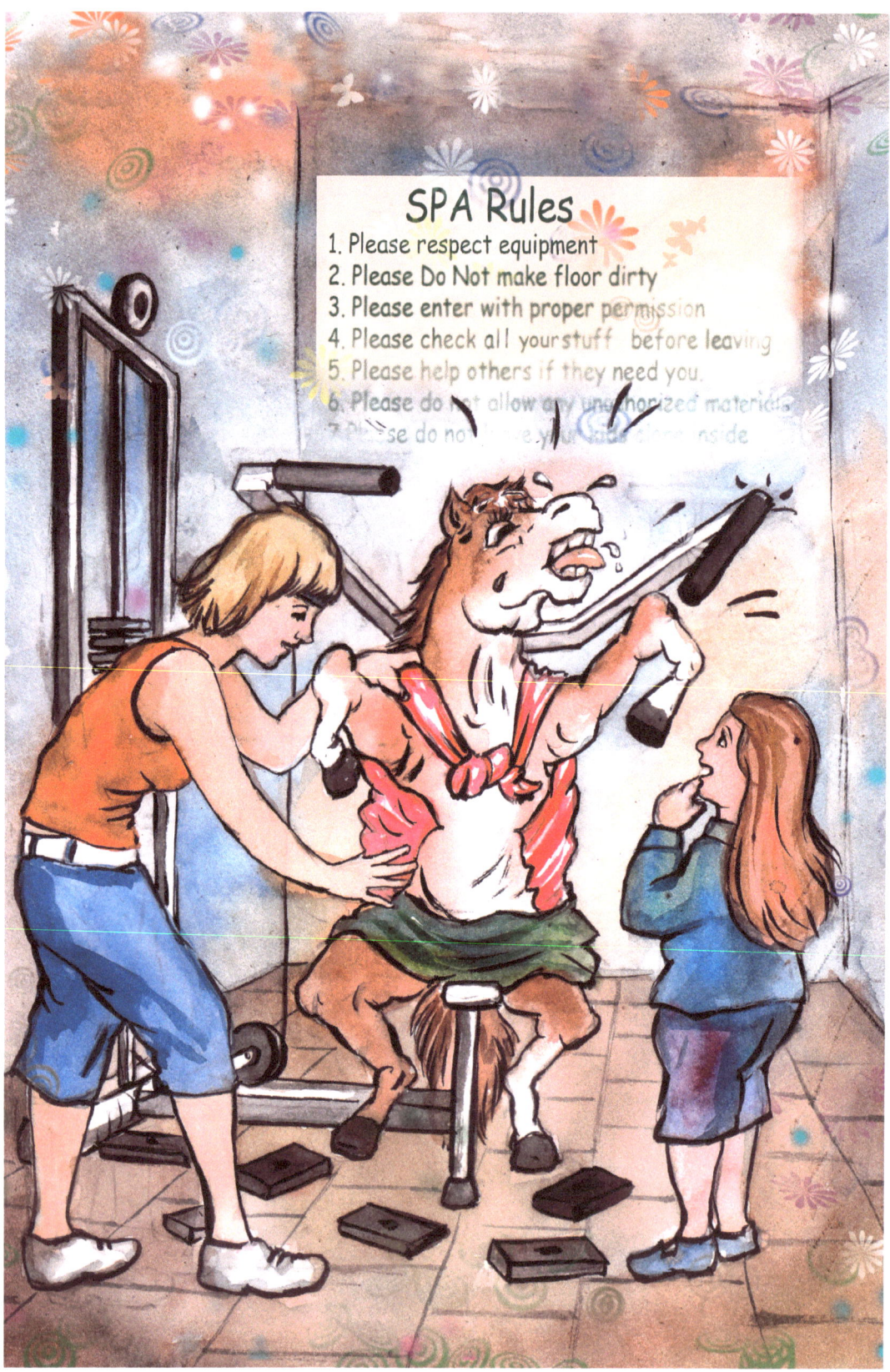

Nessie tried to open the door, but Bessie Biceps was leaning against it while talking to Tracy Triceps about Tessie. Tessie and Nessie were sweating and yelling, "Let us out of here!" Just when Nessie thought she would melt, she woke up. She was hot and sweaty but happy to be in her own bed with a sheet and covers over her instead of a towel. Tessie was nowhere to be seen and neither were any biceps or triceps or treadmills or weights. Maybe she should have skipped the pizza snack before bed and had milk or a piece of fruit.

What other kind of snacks could she have eaten before she went to bed instead of pizza so she might not have had such a nightmare?

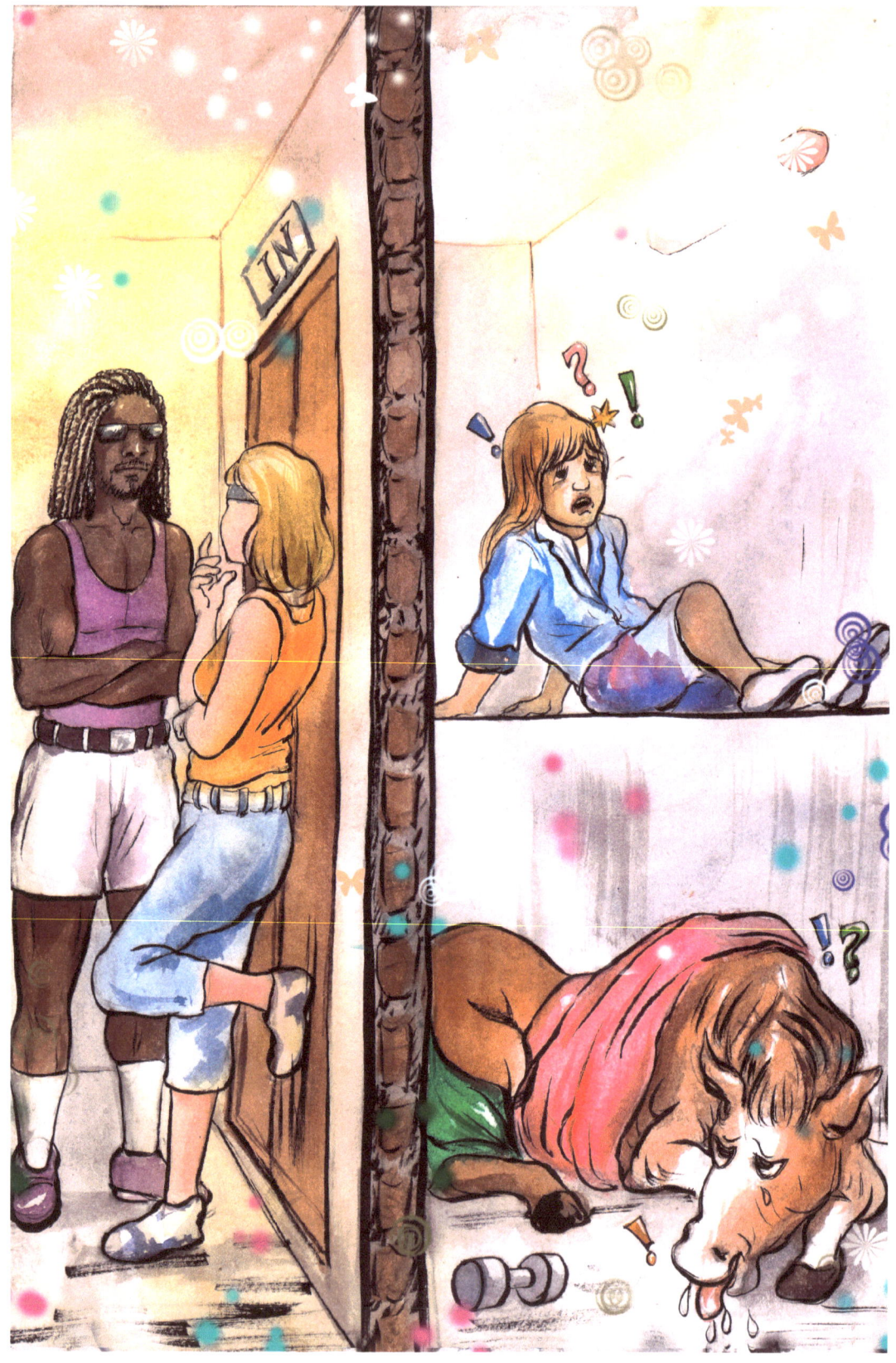

The next morning she went to meet the real Tessie at the stable. First she put a halter on Tessie and carefully led her around the arena. When Tessie's feet started to hurt, and she started to limp, Nessie took her back to the stall. She patted Tessie on the nose and said, "I'll be back tomorrow. Don't worry Tessie."

The vet came and gave Tessie more medicine and ointment. After a few weeks, Tessie's feet were better, and the riding instructor showed Nessie how to put a saddle blanket and a saddle on Tessie. She put her foot in the stirrup and swung up onto Tessie's back. She had never felt so happy. Tessie seemed to like it too. She turned her head around and looked back at Nessie on her back and whinnied. After a few more weeks, Tessie lost enough weight so that her feet didn't hurt anymore, and Nessie could ride her outside. Nessie lost weight too because she was exercising more and having so much fun that she forgot to eat so much.

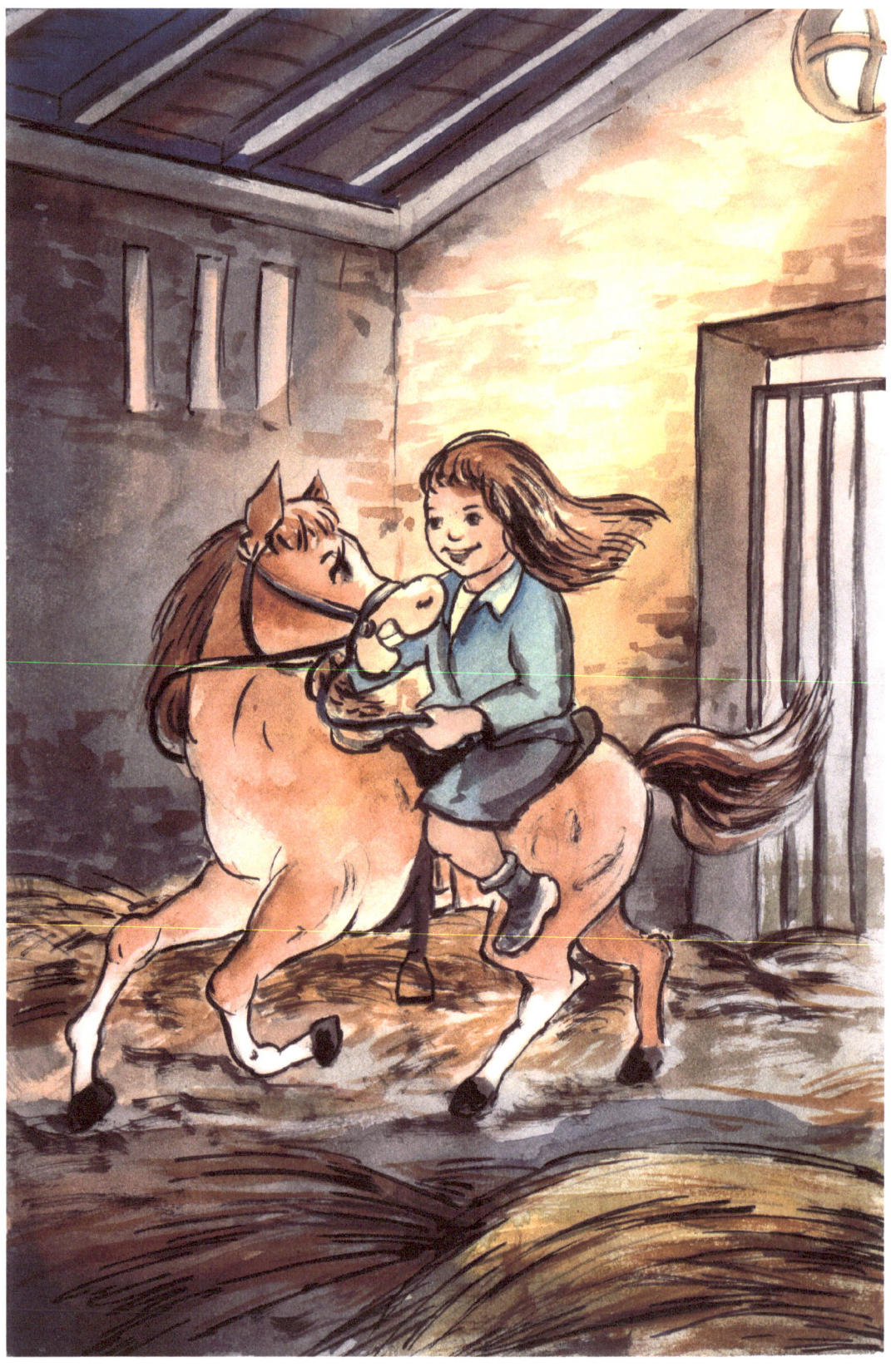

But that is not all Nessie did to lose weight and feel better. She remembered that Tessie ate grass, apples, carrots, and oats but not candy, soft drinks, or fast food. Nessie's mother had read a book about healthy eating, especially eating more fresh vegetables and fruit. She was giving the whole family several helpings of fruit and vegetables every day.

For breakfast Nessie always had a banana with her cereal. She also had an orange, a tangerine or juice like apple or grape. For lunch at home or at school she had another type of fruit such as peaches, pears or kiwi fruit. Her mother always served salads and vegetables for dinner. The whole family was feeling better and Nessie was glad. She liked broccoli the way her mother fixed it with raisins and nuts and was quite fond of apples and carrots because Tessie ate them. Her brother even seemed a little nicer after eating vegetables, but not much.

Do you eat fruit and vegetables every day?

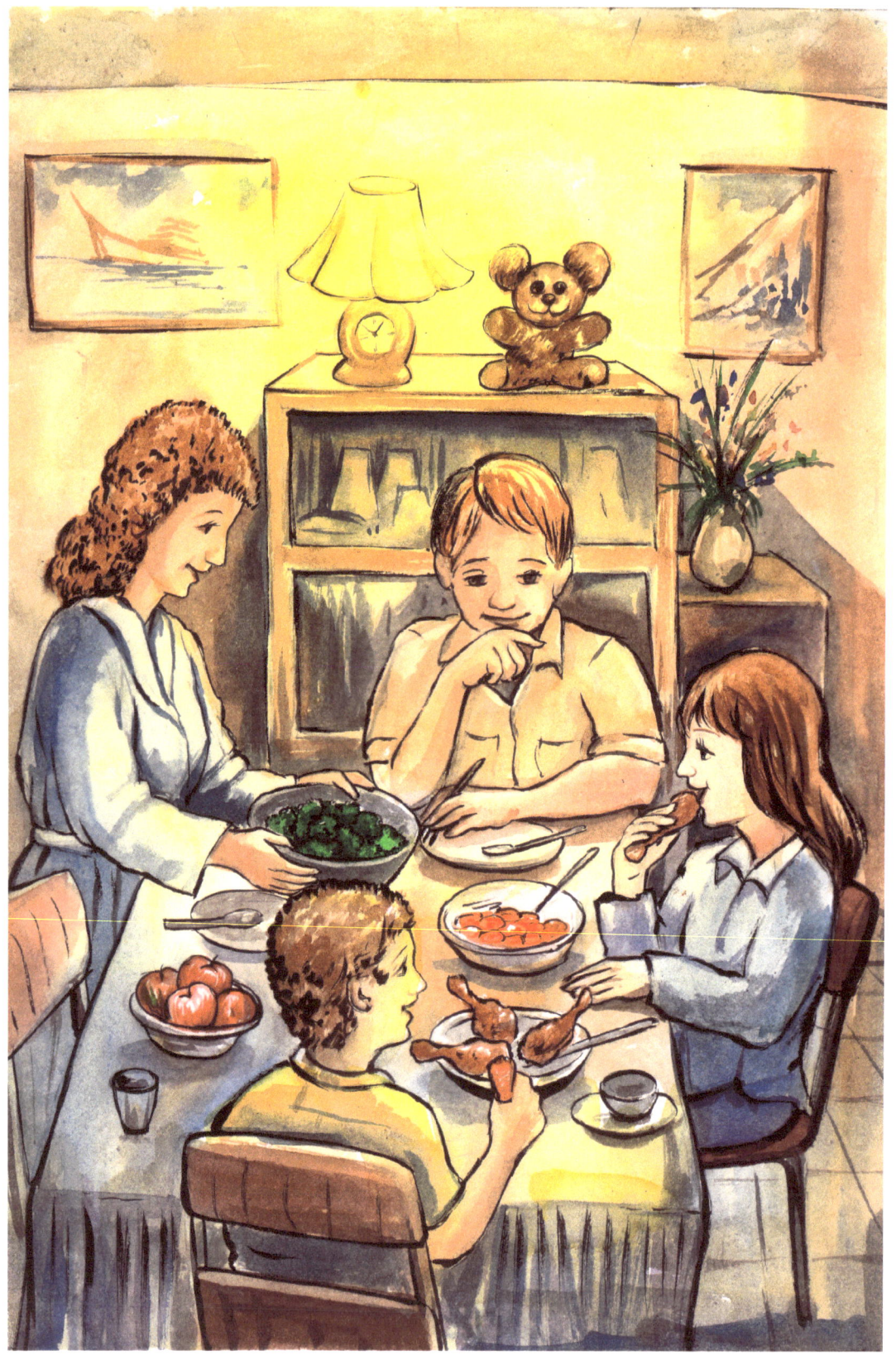

Tessie and Nessie were doing so well with their lesson, their riding instructor suggested that they enter the horse show. Nessie brushed Tessie until she was as shiny as a copper penny, and her mane and tail were beautiful. When Nessie bought a new red and black riding outfit for the show, it was the same size that she wore before she started eating too much and gaining weight. They rode into the ring and went through their different paces. They did turns, and backed up, and trotted in place. Everyone clapped and cheered when Tessie did a little dance and bowed to the crowd.

They trotted to the end of the ring and waited for the judges' decision. Nessie crossed her fingers and Tessie crossed her hooves while the judges totaled their points.

Do you think they won a prize?

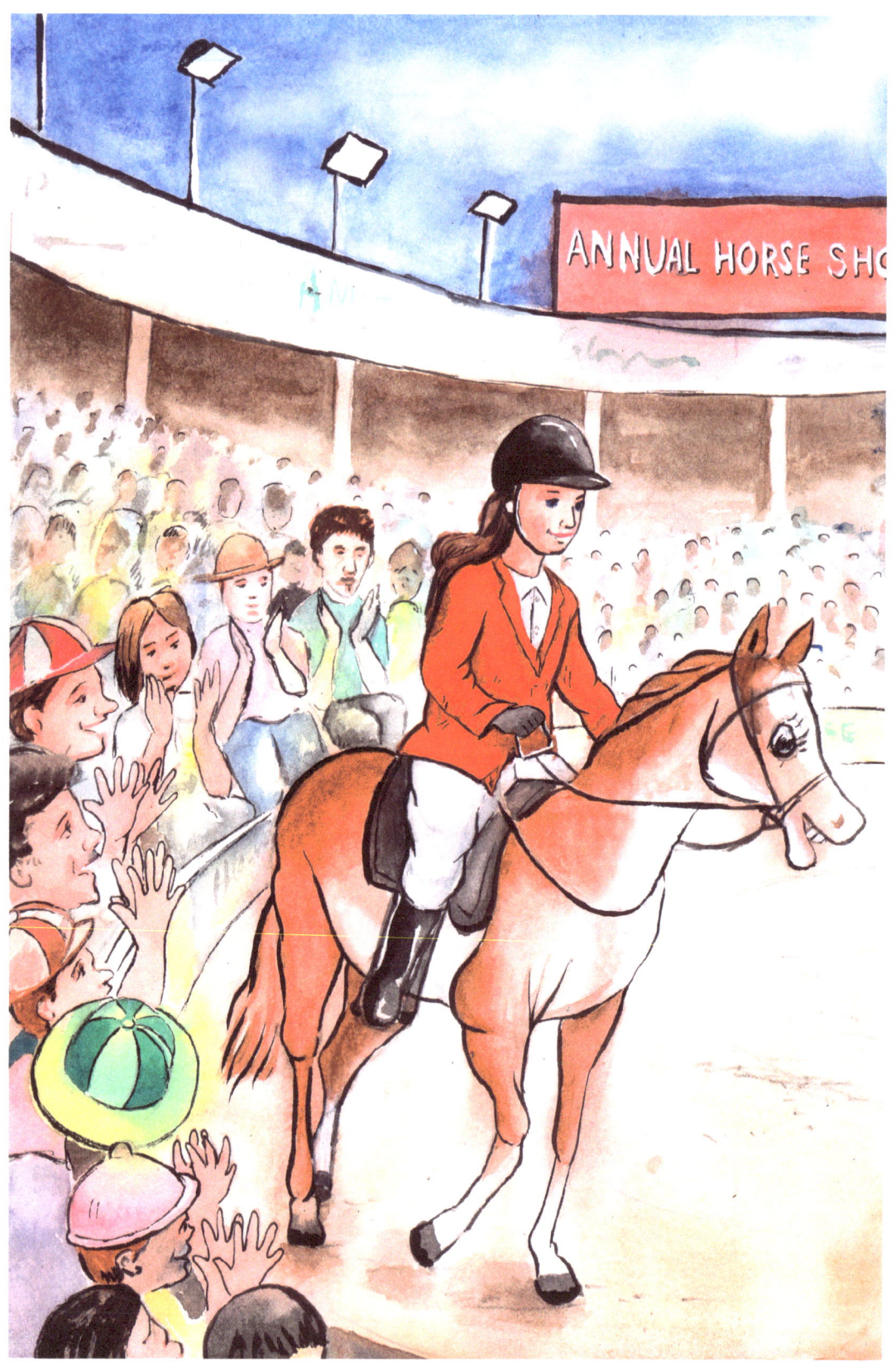

You are right if you said, "yey" because the judges awarded them the second prize, and they shouted and whinnied for joy! Nessie received a red and gold ribbon and Tessie got a red ribbon too. Her parents were very proud of them. Her brother said, "Congratulations, Vanessa!" She said, "You can call me Nessie now because it rhymes with Tessie, my new friend."

And speaking of friends, Amy, Nessie's friend who had moved away, was there to see her at the horse show and so were some of her other friends from school. The horses nodded their heads up and down to Tessie as if to congratulate her. Tessie and Nessie were not sad and lonesome anymore.

Do you think that eating right and exercising had something to do with this?

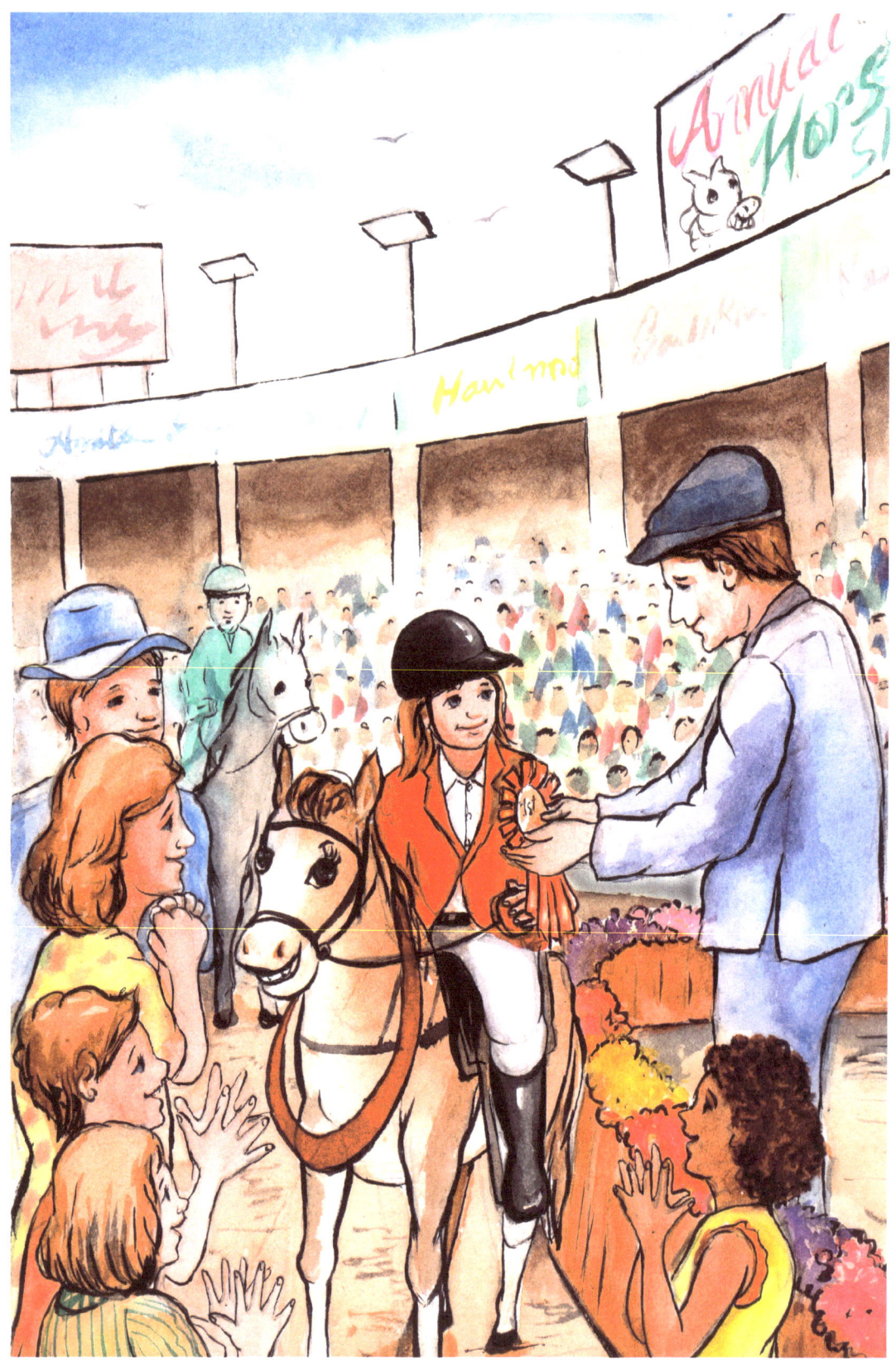

Tessie and Nessie decided to enter the horse show again the next year and try to win another prize. But they felt like winners even without a prize because they were thin and healthy again. When everyone had left, Nessie jokingly asked, "Tessie, do you want to go to the gym with me and exercise?"

Tessie put her nose in the air and said, "'Neigh' (meaning no). My jogging suit is much too big for me now."

****

Even if you don't have a horse farm near you, you can run with your friends, or walk your dog, or ride your bike or start a garden, or play tennis, football, basketball, soccer, baseball, go bowling or play with your skateboard. Can you think of more ways to stay active and have fun? Many of Nessie's friends who were not horse lovers did other things that were fun, like playing on a basketball team or hiking in the woods.

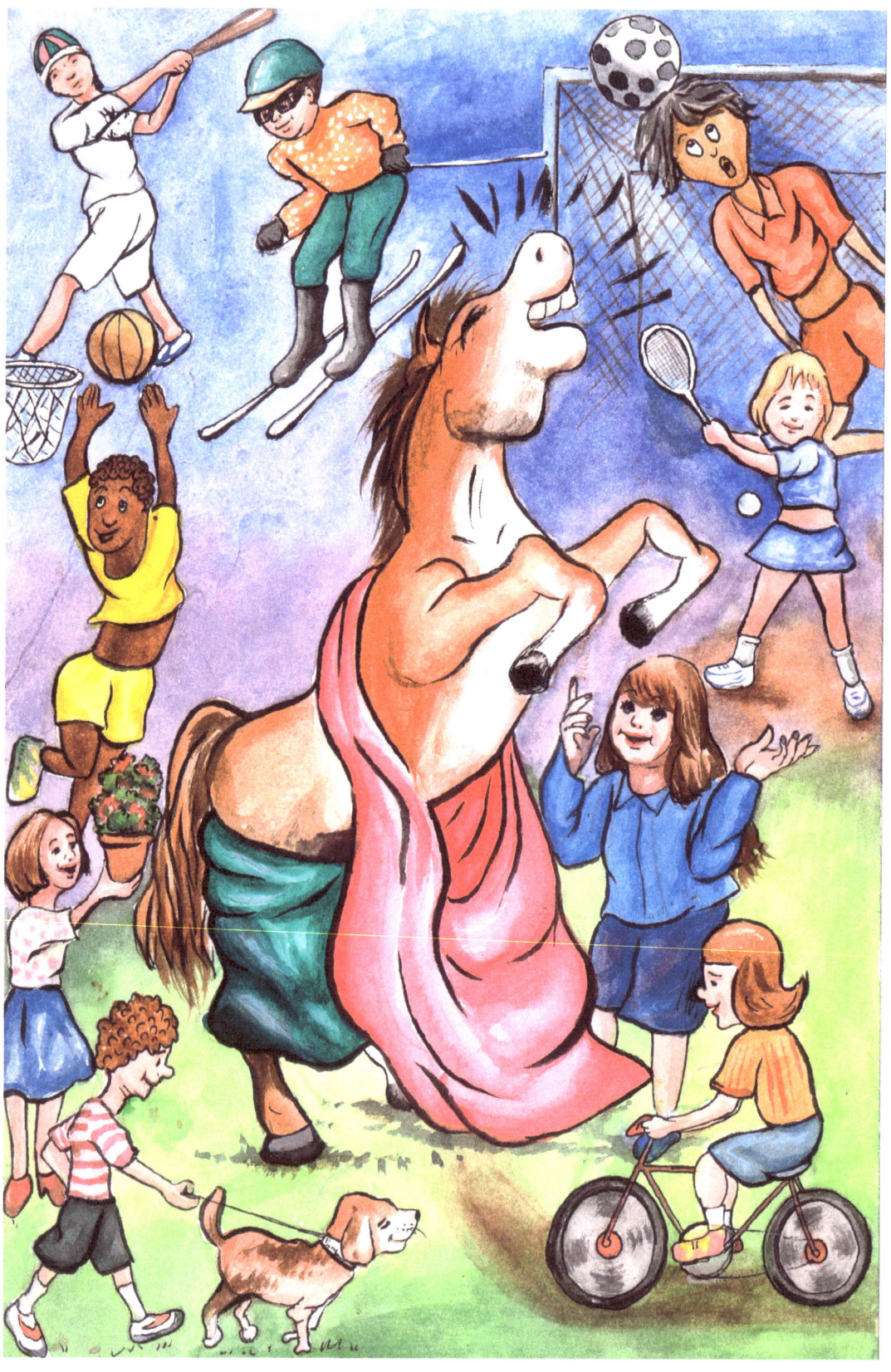

Notes for Parents: As with many conditions, a range of factors, which often act in combination, can bring on childhood obesity.

Dietary
Soft drink consumption may contribute to childhood obesity. In a study of 548 children over a 19 month period the likelihood of obesity increased by 1.6 for every increase in soft drink consumed per day

Eating at fast food restaurants has become prevalent among young people with 75% of 7 to 12 grade students consuming fast food in a given week Some literature has found a relationship between fat food consumption and obesity. Including a study which found that fast food restaurants near schools increases the risk of obesity among the student population

Whole milk consumption verses 2% milk consumption in children of one to two years of age had no effect on weight, height, or body fat percentage. Therefore whole milk continues to be recommended for this age group. However the trend of substituting sweetened drink for milk has been found to lead to excess weight gain

Sedentary lifestyle
Physical inactivity of children has also shown to be a serious cause, and children who fail to engage in regular physical activity are at greater risk of obesity. Researchers studied the physical activity of 133 children over a three-week period using an accelerometer to measure each child's level of physical activity. They discovered the obese children were 35%

less active on school days and 65% less active on weekends compared to non-obese children.

Many children fail to exercise because they are spending time doing stationary activities such as playing video games or watching TV. TV and other technology may be large factors of physically inactive children. Researchers provided a technology questionnaire to 4,561 children, ages 14, 16, and 18. They discovered children were 21.5% more likely to be overweight when watching 4+ hours of TV per day, 4.5% more likely to be overweight when using a computer one or more hours per day, and unaffected by potential weight gain from playing video games. A randomized trial showed that reducing television viewing and computer use can decrease age-adjusted BMI; reduced calorie intake was thought to be the greatest contributor to the BMI decrease.

Psychological Factors

Researchers surveyed 1,520 children, ages 9–10, with a four year follow up and discovered a positive correlation between obesity and low self esteem in the four year follow up. They also discovered that decreased self esteem led to 19% of obese children feeling sad, 48% of them feeling bored, and 21% of them feeling nervous. In comparison, 8% of normal weight children felt sad, 42% of them felt bored, and 12% of them felt nervous. Stress can also influence a child's eating habits, as can feelings of depression.

Effects on health

The first problems to occur in obese children are usually emotional or psychological. Childhood obesity however can also lead to life-threatening conditions including diabetes, high blood pressure, heart disease, sleep problems, cancer, and other disorders. Some of the other disorders would include liver disease, early puberty or menarche, eating disorders such as anorexia and bulimia, skin infections, and asthma and other respiratory problems. Studies have shown that overweight children are more likely to grow up to be overweight adults.

Obesity during adolescence has been found to increase mortality rates during adulthood. Obese children often suffer from teasing by their peers. Some are harassed or discriminated against by their own family. Stereotypes abound and may lead to low self-esteem and depression.

A 2008 study has found that children who are obese have carotid arteries which have prematurely aged by as much as thirty years as well as abnormal levels of cholesterol

Infromation from http://en.wikipedia.org/wiki/Childhood_obesity

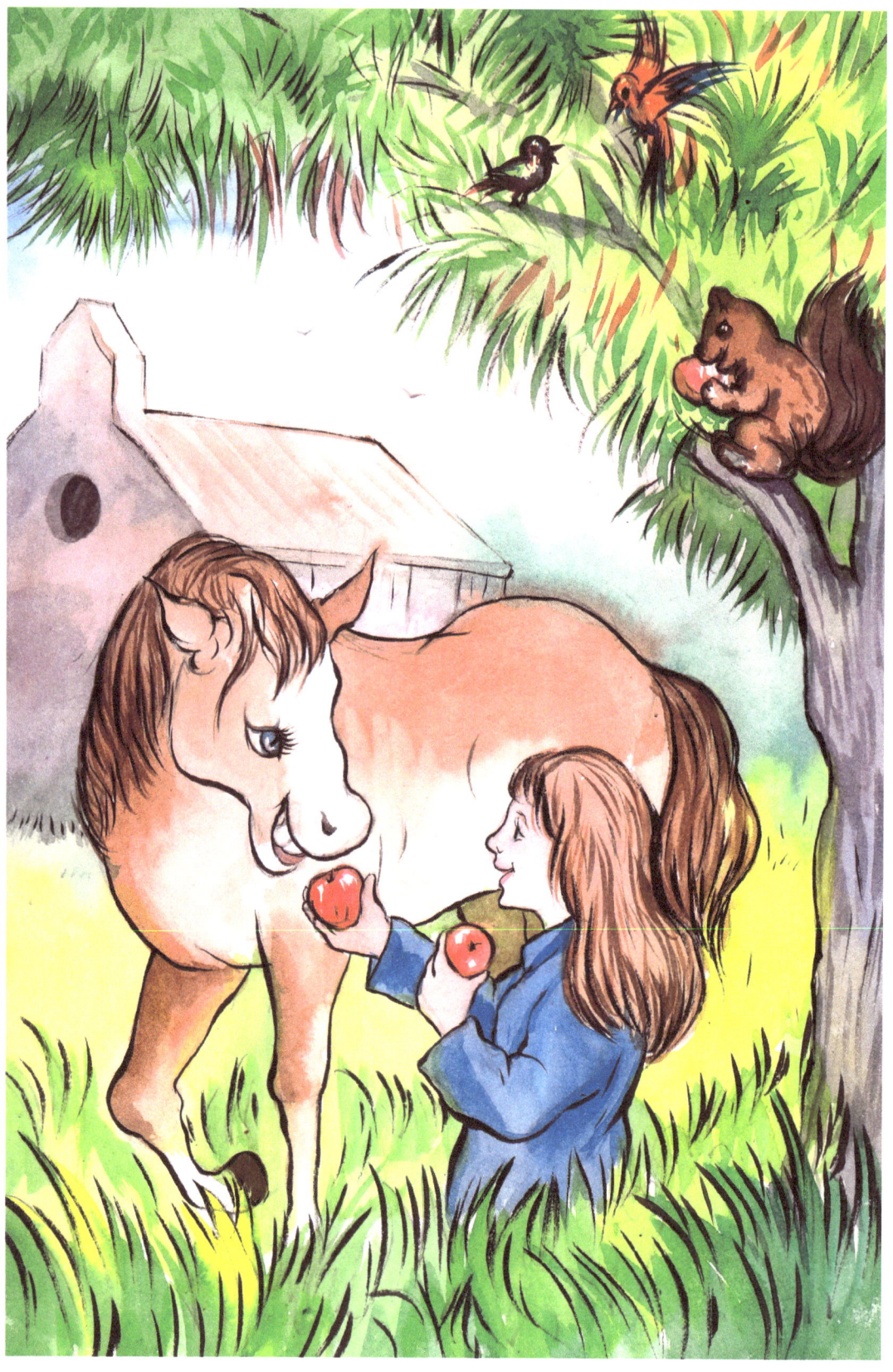